DIY
Kitchen Beauty
Recipes

L. Joy Douglas

ISBN: 149360936X
ISBN-13: 9781493609369

DEDICATION

For Rose Mary,
who I have never seen wearing any make-up.
Yet, she possesses one of the most lovely spirits
I have ever been blessed to know.

"A woman deserves no credit for beauty at sixteen,

but beauty at sixty is her soul's own doing."

CONTENTS

Disclaimer

Introduction

1   Facial Cleansers

2   Facial Scrubs

3   Facial Masks

4   Toners

5   Moisturizers

6   Eyes

7   Powders

8   Body Scrubs

9   Deodorant

10   Hair

11   Miscellaneous

Disclaimer and Copyright Information

The information found here is for informational purposes only. These recipes are the culmination of many years of research, experimentation and personal experience. I do not claim to be an expert in the formulation of beauty products, nor am I a dermatologist.

Warning: Please be aware that although the ingredients used in these recipes are completely natural, that does not mean they cannot cause negative reaction in the skin. Some individuals may have serious food allergies or skin sensitivity which could be aggravated by topical application. By reading this disclaimer, you agree that I cannot be held responsible for any negative effects resulting in the use of these recipes.

Always use a clean spatula or spoon every time you dip into these treatments. This helps prevent spoilage from exposure to bacteria.

These statements have not been evaluated by the FDA. Any products discussed are not intended to diagnose, treat, cure, or prevent any disease.

10

A NOTE FROM THE AUTHOR

My clients are always asking for tips and advice on how they can better care for their skin and hair at home. Of course, I can always recommend products from the professional lines we carry in the salon. But, the fact of the matter is, many women today are feeling the economical pinch. When it comes to beauty, they want simplicity, quality and affordability. Not everyone's budget allows for a $90 eye cream, a $30 shampoo or a $75 body scrub.

Back in the mid 90's, I ran across a book on aromatherapy. In those pages, I discovered a holistic approach to beauty treatments. There were guides on how to plant, grow and harvest your own herbs and spices, as well as suggestions on how to use essential oils. These ingredients were then combined with other natural foods to create recipes for use in home beauty regimens.

Although I cannot remember the name of that book today, the seed of an idea was planted. All through my career in the beauty industry, I have been pushed to "sell". Sell shampoo, hairspray, body cream, facial cleanser, etc. It was very difficult for me to do that because I knew that no matter how high the quality of product, retail being what it is, I was always charging too much money for products that were not the healthiest choice.

Do not misunderstand! There are some amazing product lines available through your salon professional. I use them daily and do recommend those high quality items to my own clients. But more and more, I encounter people who are looking for a more natural option when it comes to the way they care for their skin and hair.

Because of all these issues, I eventually embarked on a personal quest. My goal was to explore every possible avenue I could find in order to discover the most effective treatments for skin, hair and body that were completely natural and wouldn't break the bank.

Over the past twenty years, I have read books, done research, experimented, talked to naturopaths and tested a multitude of recipes in my own kitchen. All this was done with the goal of being able to offer people a better alternative to the high priced, chemically laden beauty products that fill the shelves today.

DIY Kitchen Beauty Recipes is the culmination of those years of collecting and experimenting. Each recipe found here has been tried by either myself, friends, or the people who created the recipes and passed them along to me.

Always remember that true beauty stems from good health. Drink water, eat fresh unprocessed foods and get moderate sun exposure. Exercise regularly and sleep well. Avoid stress! Take time to pray and practice generosity. Begin each day with gratitude. Then, incorporate some of the recipes you will find here. It is my hope that you too will discover the joys of a holistic beauty regimen, and uncover your own personal radiance!

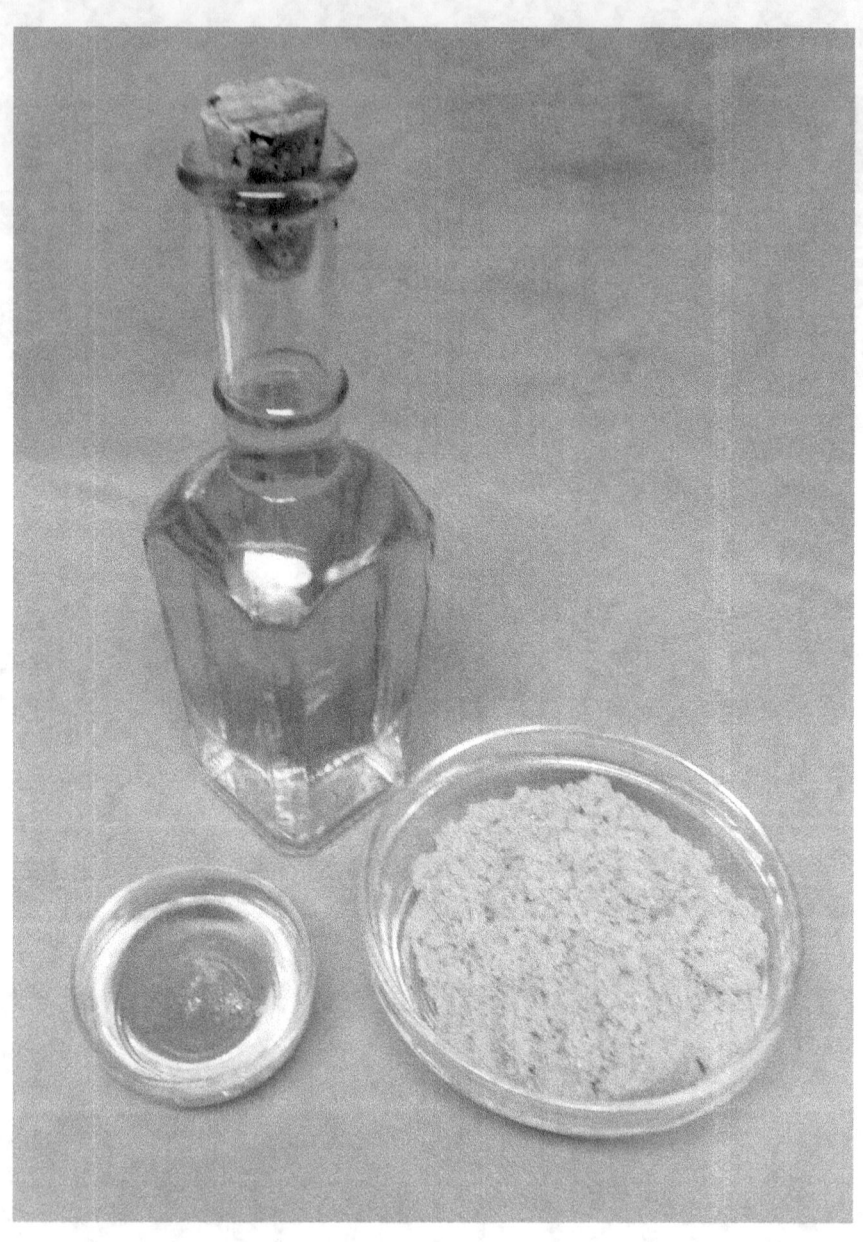

FACIAL CLEANSERS

Brightening Cleanser

Ingredients:

2 Tbsp. raw honey

1 Tbsp. plain Greek yogurt

1 Tbsp. sour cream

1 Tbsp. lemon juice

Instructions:

Mix ingredients together and apply to damp skin. Massage gently. Rinse with warm, then cool water. (optional: leave on for 15 minutes as a mask)

Strawberry Acne Cleanser

Ingredients:

3 large strawberries (mashed)

2 Tbsp. plain Greek yogurt

½ tsp. lemon juice

Instructions:

Mix all ingredients together and apply liberally to damp skin. Massage gently in a circular motion. Rinse well with warm water and pat dry. Follow with natural moisturizer.

Citrus Aloe Cleanser

Ingredients:

¼ C. aloe vera gel

1 tsp. liquid castile soap

2 tsp. almond oil

25-30 drops orange essential oil

Instructions:

Combine all ingredients in a jar or bottle. Stir to mix. Place cap on container and shake vigorously, ensuring a complete blend of ingredients. Apply small amount to damp skin and massage gently all over face and neck. Rinse well with warm, then cool water. Pat dry and follow with natural moisturizer.

Exfoliating Honey Cleanser

Ingredients:

1 Tbsp. raw honey

½ tsp. baking soda

½ tsp. water

Instructions:

Combine ingredients together to form a paste. Massage gently into damp skin and rinse completely with warm water. Follow with a light application of natural moisturizer.

Gentle Oatmeal Wash

(Save back a spoonful of breakfast to make this one!)

Ingredients:

1 Tbsp. oatmeal (cooked)

1 Tbsp. plain Greek yogurt

1 tsp. raw honey

Instructions:

Apply to damp skin, massaging gently for 30 seconds. Rinse well with warm , then cool water. Pat dry and apply moisturizer

----

Oil Cleanser

Ingredients:

1 tsp. castor oil

1 tsp. extra virgin olive oil

Instructions:

Mix oils together and apply to face, massaging gently but thoroughly for 2 minutes. Soak a washcloth in hot water, wring out excess and hold cloth to face for 30 seconds. As the cloth cools down, wipe off some of the oil. Repeat several times until the oil has been rinsed away. Finish with a cool washcloth.

Soothing Almond Cleanser

Ingredients:

2 Tbsp. plain Greek yogurt

1 tsp. raw honey

1 tsp. almond oil

Instructions:

Mix together yogurt, honey and almond oil in a small bowl. Apply to damp skin, massaging gently. Rinse well with warm water.

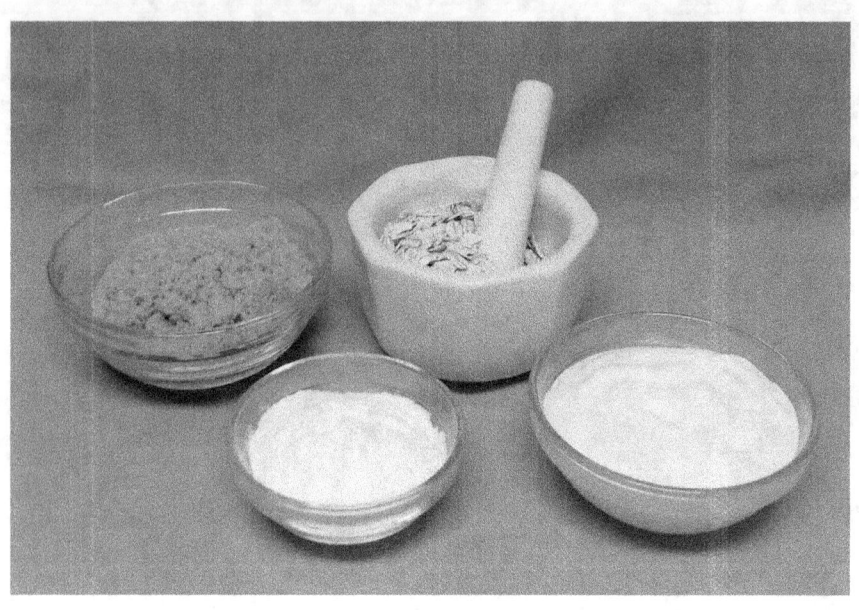

FACIAL SCRUBS

Oatmeal-Lavender Face Scrub

Ingredients:

1 C. oatmeal

1/2 C. cornmeal

1/2 C. powdered milk

2 tsp. brown sugar

3 Tbsp. plain yogurt

5 drops lavender essential oil

Instructions:

Mix all the dry ingredients together. Stir in yogurt and oil. Massage gently into freshly cleansed skin. Rinse with warm water. (Can also be used as a body exfoliant.)

Citrus Facial Scrub

Ingredients:

1 Tbsp. dried citrus peel (orange, lemon, lime or grapefruit)

½ C. plain yogurt

1 tsp. raw honey

¼ C. almond oil or vitamin E oil

1 Tbsp. brown sugar

1 Tbsp. cornmeal

Instructions:

Grind citrus peel in food processor. Add remaining ingredients and mix well. Apply to freshly cleansed skin and massage gently in circular motion. Rinse with cool water.

Honey Oat Facial Scrub

Ingredients:

1 Tbsp. oatmeal

I Tbsp. brown sugar

1 Tbsp. ground almonds

1 Tbsp. raw honey

1 Tbsp. plain Greek yogurt

Instructions:

Combine dry ingredients in a bowl. Stir in honey and yogurt to mix well. Apply to freshly cleansed skin and massage gently in a circular motion. Rinse well with warm water.

Coffee Sugar Scrub

Ingredients:

½ C. sugar

½ C. ground coffee

¼ C. coconut oil, melted

¼ cup jojoba or almond oil

10 drops vanilla

Instructions:

Mix all ingredients to form a paste. Apply to freshly cleansed skin and massage in a circular motion. Rinse with warm water.

Honey Vanilla Skin Polisher

Ingredients:

1 C. brown sugar

¼ C. coconut oil, melted

¼ C. almond oil or jojoba oil

¼ C. raw honey

10 drops vanilla

Instructions:

Mix all ingredients to form a paste. Apply to freshly cleansed skin and massage gently in circular motion. Leave on as a mask for 5 minutes and rinse well, first with warm, then cool water.

Bee Gorgeous

Ingredients:

2 Tbsp. raw honey

2 Tbsp. almond oil or coconut oil (melted)

2 Tbsp. ground flax seeds

3 Tbsp. brown sugar

Instructions:

Mix all ingredients together in a bowl. Apply to freshly cleansed skin and massage gently in a circular motion. Rinse well with warm water.

Blackhead Busting Exfoliator:

Ingredients:

1 Tbsp. sugar

1 Tbsp. baking soda

2 Tbsp. warm water

Instructions:

Mix all ingredients together in a bowl. Apply to freshly cleansed skin and massage gently in a circular motion. Rinse well with warm water. Pat dry and apply a thin layer of coconut oil or other natural moisturizer.

Gentle Skin Polish

Ingredients:

1 tsp. coconut oil

½ tsp. baking soda

Instructions:

Cleanse face and leave skin damp. Place both ingredients in the palm of one hand and mix together with hands. Apply to face and gently massage into skin using a circular motion. Rinse well with warm water and pat dry. No need to use moisturizer. The coconut oil will leave a thin protective barrier and leave your skin silky smooth. (This is my "go to" recipe for a quick, gentle and effective exfoliator!)

Cinnamon Lip Scrub

Ingredients:

½ tsp. sugar

½ tsp. raw honey

½ tsp. almond oil

2-3 shakes cinnamon

Instructions:

Mix all ingredients together. Gently massage into lips with fingertip using a circular motion. Rinse well with warm water. Pat dry and seal in moisture with a thin layer of almond oil or natural lip balm.

Gentle Acne Scrub

Ingredients:

2 Tbsp. brown sugar

½ tsp. olive oil

5 drops thyme essential oil

Instructions:

Mix all ingredients together. Apply to cleansed skin in sweeping, upward motions. Rinse well with warm water and pat dry. Follow with a thin layer of coconut oil or other natural moisturizer.

Simple Scrub

Ingredients:

1 tsp. baking soda

1 Tbsp. raw honey

Instructions:

Combine ingredients to form a paste. Apply to freshly cleansed skin and massage gently using circular motions. Rinse well with warm water and pat dry. Follow with a thin layer of natural moisturizer. This is gentle enough to be used a few times a week.

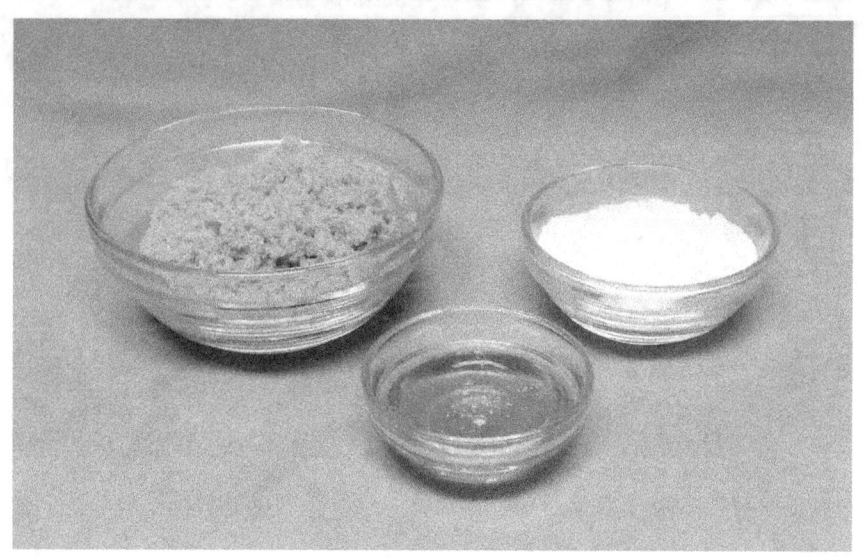

FACIAL MASKS

Berry Yogurt Mask

Ingredients:

2 Tbsp. plain Greek yogurt

2 Tbsp. raw honey

¼ C. berries (black berries, strawberries, raspberries, etc.)

1 tsp. lemon juice

½ tsp. apple cider vinegar

Instructions:

Pulse yogurt and honey in blender until combined. Add berries and puree. Add lemon juice and vinegar and blend until well mixed. Apply generously to clean skin (avoiding eye area) and let sit for 15 minutes. Rinse well with warm water and pat dry. Follow with natural moisturizer.

Classic Egg White Tightening Mask

Ingredients:

1 egg white

Instructions:

Apply egg white to freshly cleansed skin with a cotton pad. Allow to dry on the face for 15 minutes. Rinse well with warm water. Pat dry. (It is recommended to follow with witch hazel toner and a light, natural moisturizer.)

Classic Egg Yolk Hydrating Mask

Ingredients:

1 egg yolk

1 tsp. raw honey

Instructions:

Mix ingredients thoroughly in a bowl using a whisk. Apply evenly to freshly cleansed skin with fingertips. Let sit for 15 minutes. Rinse well with warm water.

Mocha Mask

Ingredients:

¼ C. ground coffee

¼ C. cocoa powder

½ C. heavy cream

Instructions:

Combine ingredients to form a paste. Apply liberally to clean skin (avoiding eye area). Let sit for 15 minutes. Rinse well with warm water. Pat dry. Moisturize.

Balancing Mask

Ingredients:

2 Tbsp. raw honey

1 Tbsp. lemon juice

Instructions:

Mix ingredients together and apply to clean skin. Let sit 15 minutes. Rinse well with warm, then cool water.

Nourishing Oatmeal Mask

Ingredients:

1 egg yolk

½ tsp. lemon juice

2 Tbsp. dry oatmeal

½ tsp. almond oil

Instructions:

Whisk egg yolk in a bowl. Add lemon juice, oatmeal and almond oil. Mix well and apply with fingertips to clean skin. Let sit 10-15 minutes. Rinse well with warm water. Pat dry.

Avocado Moisture Treatment

Ingredients:

1 ripe avocado

1 Tbsp. olive oil

2 tsp. lemon juice

Instructions:

Cut avocado in half and discard the pit. Scoop out flesh into a bowl and mash well. Add oil and lemon juice and mix thoroughly. Apply generously to freshly cleansed skin, smoothing over entire face. Let sit for 15 minutes. Rinse well with warm water.

Clearing Mask (for acne)

Ingredients:

3 tsp. raw honey

½ tsp. cinnamon

Instructions:

Mix ingredients together. Apply to skin with fingertips. Let sit for 15-20 minutes. Rinse well with warm, then cool water. Pat dry.------------

Moisture Mask (for dry skin)

Ingredients:

1 tsp. raw honey

1 tsp. plain Greek yogurt

½ avocado (mashed)

Instructions:

Place ingredients in a bowl and beat with hand mixer until smooth. Apply to freshly cleansed skin with fingertips and let sit for 15-20 minutes. Rinse well with warm water and pat dry. Follow with a thin layer of coconut oil or a few drops of vitamin E oil.

Redness Reducer

Ingredients:

1 pickling size cucumber (*not* an actual pickle!)

1 egg white

1 Tbsp. raw honey

½ C. oatmeal

½ tsp. baking soda

Instructions:

Puree cucumber and egg white in blender. Place in a bowl and stir in remaining ingredients. Apply paste with fingertips to clean skin and allow to dry up to 30 minutes. Wet a cloth with warm water. Wring out excess and place over face to soften mask. When the cloth has cooled, wipe off mask. Follow by rinsing skin with warm, then cool water. Pat dry and apply a few drops of vitamin E oil.

Tightening Mask

Ingredients:

1 Tbsp. raw honey

1 Tbsp. plain Greek yogurt

1 Tbsp. espresso grounds

Instructions:

Combine ingredients to form a paste. Apply a thick layer to clean skin with fingertips or cosmetic spatula. Let sit for 10 -15 minutes and rinse thoroughly with warm water. Follow with a splash of cold water.

Sweet Spice Mask (for acne prone dry skin)

Ingredients:

½ tsp. heavy cream

½ tsp. raw honey

¼ tsp. cinnamon

¼ tsp. nutmeg

Instructions:

Mix ingredients in a small bowl. Apply to freshly cleansed skin and massage gently, avoiding eye area. Leave mask on for 20 minutes and then rinse well with warm water. Follow with a few drops of vitamin E or coconut oil.

Wrinkle Fighter

Ingredients:

½ small cucumber, peeled and seeded

1 tsp. lemon juice

1 egg white

Instructions:

Peel cucumber, discard seeds and chop into chunks. Place in blender with remaining ingredients and puree. Apply to clean skin with a cotton ball. Let sit for 15 minutes and rinse well with warm water. Follow with a splash of cold water. Pat dry and finish with a few drops of almond oil to soften.

Chocolate Mask

Ingredients:

¼ C. cocoa powder

2 Tbsp. oatmeal

3 Tbsp. raw honey

¼ C. heavy cream

5 drops vanilla

Instructions:

Place first two ingredients in a bowl and mix with fork. Add wet ingredients and whip with hand mixer. Apply to clean skin in a thick, even layer and leave on for 10 minutes.
 (Yes, it is okay to taste the leftovers!) Rinse well with warm water and pat skin dry.

Healing Treatment Mask

Ingredients:

1 Tbsp. sour cream

1 Tbsp. plain Greek yogurt

2 Tbsp. raw honey

1 Tbsp. apple cider vinegar

Instructions:

Place all ingredients in a bowl and combine with a whisk. Apply to clean skin and let sit for 15-20 minutes. Rinse with warm, then cool water. Pat dry and follow with a light, natural moisturizer.

Soothing Gel Mask (for sensitive skin)

Ingredients:

1 tsp. aloe vera gel

2 tsp. raw honey

Instructions:

Combine ingredients by stirring together. Smooth over clean skin and leave for 15 minutes. Rinse with warm water and pat dry. Follow with a few drops of vitamin E oil.

Natural Botox Alternative

Ingredients:

½ ripe banana

¾ C. plain Greek yogurt

1 Tbsp. raw honey

Instructions:

Mash banana and stir in remaining ingredients. Apply a generous layer over cleansed skin. Wet a clean cloth with warm water and wring out excess. Recline and relax, placing cloth over face for 15 minutes. Remove mask with cloth and follow by rinsing thoroughly. Pat dry.

Restoring Mask

Ingredients:

Flesh of one ripe avocado

1 egg yolk

2 Tbsp. raw honey

1 tsp. plain Greek yogurt

1 Tbsp. avocado oil

Instructions:

Combine all the ingredients with a hand mixer until smooth. Cleanse skin with very warm water and pat dry. Immediately apply mask and let sit for 15 minutes. Remove with damp cotton pads or warm washcloth. Rinse thoroughly with warm, then cool water.

Antioxidant Treatment

Ingredients:

15 fresh blueberries

1 Tbsp. raw honey

1 Tbsp. heavy cream

Instructions:

Mash berries in a bowl with your hands (wear gloves to avoid staining fingers). Mix in honey and cream with a whisk. Apply generously to clean skin and let sit 15 minutes. Rinse with warm water. Pat dry and apply a thin layer of coconut oil or light weight, natural moisturizer.

Pineapple Soothing Treatment

½ C. crushed pineapple (drained)

1 egg yolk

1 Tbsp. heavy cream

1 Tbsp. almond oil

3 Tbsp. almond meal/flour

Instructions:

Place first four ingredients in blender and puree. Stir in almond flour to form a paste. Apply to clean skin and let sit for 15 minutes. Rinse well with warm water and pat dry.

Firming Facial Mask

Ingredients:

1 egg white (chilled)

1 tsp. cornstarch

Instructions:

Whisk ingredients together until smooth and airy. Spread a thin layer onto clean skin with fingers. Recline and relax, allowing mask to dry for 20 minutes. Rinse thoroughly with warm water and pat skin dry. Finish with the application of natural moisturizer.

Brightening Mask

Ingredients:

1 large slice ripe papaya

Instructions:

Discard seeds and separate pulp from peel. Wash face with warm water and gentle cleanser and pat dry. Rub the inside of the papaya peel all over face and let dry 15 minutes. Rinse well and pat dry. Apply a few drops of vitamin E oil.

Clear Complexion Mask

Ingredients:

1 Tbsp. orange juice

1 Tbsp. baking soda

Instructions:

Stir ingredients together until fizzing subsides. Dip cotton ball in solution and sweep over face. Let sit for 15-20 minutes. Rinse well and pat dry. Apply light weight moisturizer.

Pumpkin Mask (for oily skin)

Ingredients:

4 Tbsp. pure pumpkin (fresh or canned)

2 Tbsp. raw honey

2 Tbsp. heavy cream

Instructions:

Spread a generous layer over freshly cleansed skin. Let sit for 10 minutes, rinse well with warm water and pat dry.-------------------------

Restorative Skin Treatment

Ingredients:

1 ripe banana

1 avocado

1 Tbsp. almond butter

1 Tbsp. raw honey

1 tsp. olive oil

1 Tbsp. orange juice

Instructions:

Puree all ingredients in blender. Apply a thick layer to clean skin. Let sit for 15 minutes or until mask begins to "draw" and tighten. Remove with a damp cloth and then rinse thoroughly with warm water. Pat dry and finish with a few drops of oil or natural moisturizer.

Chocolate Moisture Treatment

Ingredients:

½ C. cocoa powder

1 Tbsp. oatmeal

¼ C. raw honey

3 Tbsp. heavy cream

2 tsp. cottage cheese or ricotta

Instructions:

Combine cocoa and oatmeal in a bowl. Add remaining ingredients and stir to mix well. Apply a generous layer to clean skin and let sit for 10 minutes. Rinse well with warm water. Pat dry.

Orange Moisture Mask

Ingredients:

¾ C. oatmeal

2 tsp. orange zest

3 Tbsp. plain Greek yogurt

2 Tbsp. raw honey

¼ C. orange juice

Instructions:

Combine oatmeal and orange zest in a bowl. Stir in remaining ingredients. Smooth a generous layer onto clean skin (avoiding eye area). Let sit for 20 minutes. Rinse well with warm, then cool water. Pat dry and apply a few drops of almond oil.

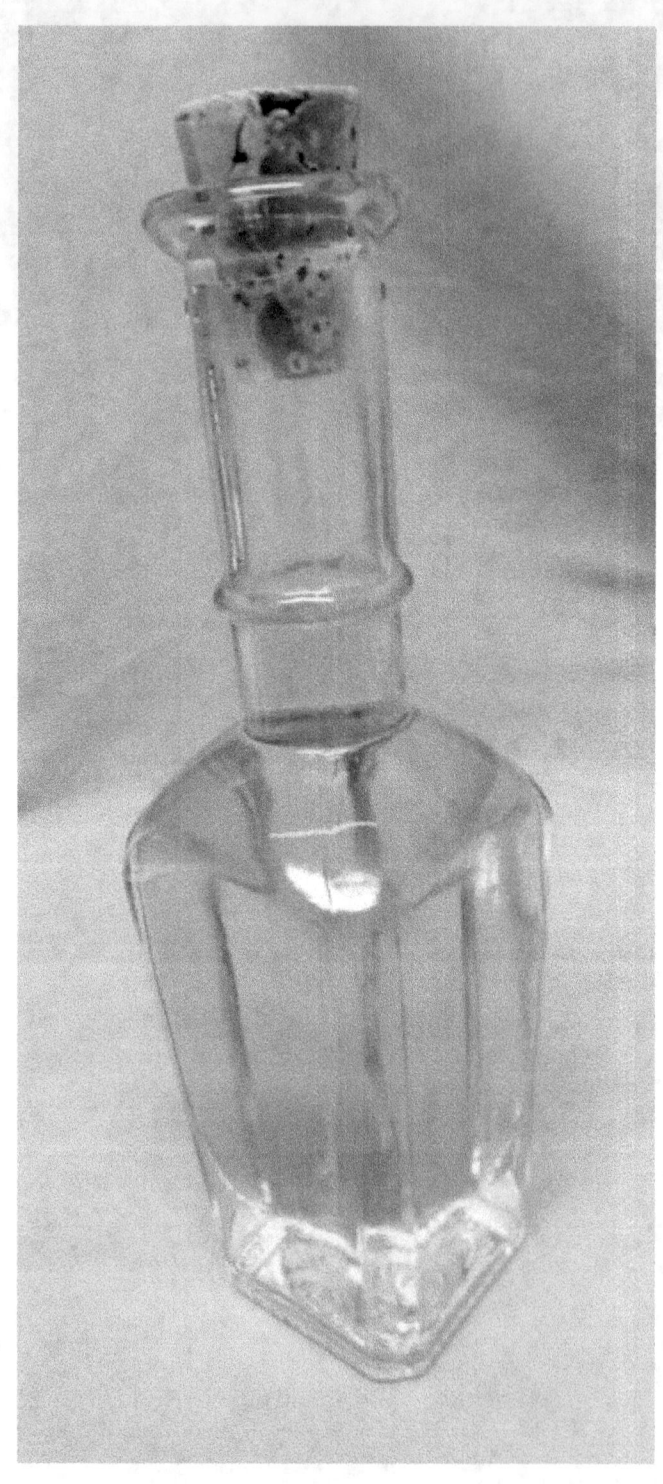

TONERS

Freshening Toner

Ingredients:

½ C. witch hazel

3 Tbsp. lemon juice

Instructions:

Combine ingredients in a bottle and shake well. Apply to freshly cleansed skin with a cotton pad. Air dry skin and apply moisturizer.

Apple Cider Toner (for acne prone skin)

Ingredients:

½ oz. apple cider vinegar

2 oz. water

3 plain uncoated aspirin tablets

Instructions:

Combine water and vinegar in a bottle. Dissolve aspirin in mixture and shake to blend. Apply toner to clean skin with a cotton pad. Follow with oil free moisturizer.

Herbal Tea Toner (for sensitive skin)

Ingredients:

1 C. filtered water

1 chamomile tea bag

Instructions:

Brew a cup of chamomile tea and allow it to cool. Apply toner to clean skin with a cotton pad. Follow with a thin layer of vitamin E.

Hydrating Facial Mist

Ingredients:

¼ C. distilled water

2 Tbsp. orange flower water

2 Tbsp. rose water

2 Tbsp. aloe vera gel

Instructions:

Combine all ingredients in a spray bottle. Mist face after cleansing or anytime you need a burst of freshness.

Tea Tree Oil Toner (for oily skin)

Ingredients:

¼ C. witch hazel

¼ C. vodka

¼ tsp. tea tree oil

Instructions:

Combine all ingredients in a bottle. Shake well to mix. Apply to freshly washed skin with a cotton pad. Follow with moisturizer.

Balancing Toner (for combination skin)

Ingredients:

1 C. distilled water

3 bags green tea

2 Tbsp. apple cider vinegar

1 Tbsp. witch hazel

1/2 Tbsp. lemon juice

2 drops almond oil

2 drops tea tree oil

Instructions:

Brew tea and allow to cool. Combine 4 Tbsp. tea with remaining ingredients. Pour mixture into bottle and shake well. Apply to clean skin with cotton pad. Store in refrigerator and shake before each use to ensure the ingredients are well blended.

Daily Toner (for acne prone skin)

Ingredients:

2 oz. distilled water

6 drops thyme oil

7 drops lavender essential oil

Instructions:

Mix ingredients together in a small glass jar and shake well to incorporate. Apply to clean skin with cotton using even strokes (avoid eye area).

Oatmeal Toner (for sensitive skin)

Ingredients:

1 packet plain instant oatmeal

hot water (use amount required on package)

Instructions:

Pour oatmeal in a glass bowl. Pour hot water into bowl, stir and allow to cook. Pour mixture through strainer and set liquid aside to cool. Apply to clean skin with cotton pad and follow with moisturizer. Pour into a bottle and store in the refrigerator for 4-5 days.

Vitamin C Toner

Ingredients:

¼ C. aloe vera juice

¼ C. witch hazel

20 drops lavender essential oil

8 drops tea tree essential oil

¼ tsp. vitamin C powder

Instructions:

Funnel all ingredients into a bottle. Place lid on tightly and shake well to combine. Apply solution to cotton ball or pad and sweep across cleansed skin.

Anti-Acne Toner

Ingredients:

1 C. green tea

¼ C. raw apple cider vinegar

2 Tbsp. aloe vera juice (*not* gel)

20 drops orange essential oil

Instructions:

Mix all ingredients in glass jar or bottle and close lid. Shake thoroughly to blend well. Apply to cotton pad and sweep over cleansed skin. Store in refrigerator.

Rice Water Toner

Ingredients:

½ C. organic rice

1 C. hot water

Instructions:

Place rice in a bowl and cover with hot water. Stir until water becomes cloudy. Allow to cool and strain water into a bottle, discarding rice. Apply to cotton ball and sweep over freshly cleansed skin. Store in refrigerator.

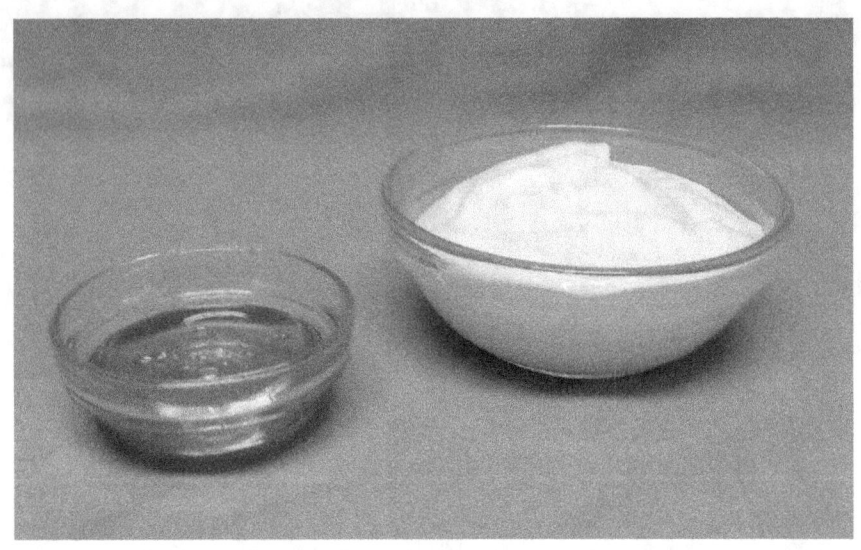

MOISTURIZERS

Coco-Mint Body Whip

Ingredients:

½ C. cocoa butter

½ C. coconut oil

20 drops peppermint essential oil

Instructions:

Place coconut oil and cocoa butter in a large bowl. Add peppermint oil and whip together with a hand mixer on low to medium. Be patient! It can take up to 10 minutes to achieve a nice, whipped consistency. (You can also use a stand mixer if you have one. It will cut down on the time by a couple of minutes.) Transfer cream to a glass jar. Apply to clean skin.

Shea & Aloe Skin Cream

Ingredients:

½ C. shea butter

2 Tbsp. coconut oil

1 Tbsp. raw honey

¼ C. aloe vera gel

5 drops tea tree oil

3 drops Vitamin E oil

Instructions:

Place water in the bottom of a double boiler. Bring to a boil and then reduce to a simmer. Melt shea butter and coconut oil. Stir in honey. Remove from heat and mix in aloe. Allow to cool for ½ hour and then stir in remaining ingredients. Transfer to a glass jar and put in the refrigerator for 3 hours. Take out of fridge, and store in a dark cabinet or drawer. Apply to clean skin, daily.

Citrus Body Butter

Ingredients:

1½ cups of coconut oil (solid)

3 Tbsp. raw honey

1 Tbsp. citrus zest (lime, lemon, orange, grapefruit)

10 drops citrus essential oil

Instructions:

Combine all ingredients in a bowl and mix well until smooth. Transfer to a glass jar. Apply to clean skin.

Natural Facial Moisturizer

Ingredients:

1/2 C. coconut oil

1 1/4 C. cocoa butter

4 Tbsp. olive oil

10 drops lavender essential oil (or oil of choice)

Instructions:

Combine all ingredients in a saucepan and heat on low until liquified. Remove from heat and allow to cool for 10 minutes. Pour into jar and cover tightly with lid. Shake the jar for 30 seconds and then let mixture settle. Shake again and place in the refrigerator to let the blend solidify. Apply to cleansed face morning and evening.

Rosemary Mint Body Butter

Ingredients:

1 ½ Tbsp. shea butter

1 ½ Tbsp. mint infused coconut oil

1 Tbsp. olive oil

2 sprigs fresh rosemary *or* 1 tsp. dried rosemary

½ tsp. vitamin E oil

5 drops lime essential oil

5 drops lavender essential oil

3 drops peppermint essential oil

Instructions:

Melt shea butter and coconut oil in a double boiler. Add olive oil and herbs. Heat mixture on low for 15 minutes. Remove from heat, strain mixture into a mixing bowl and discard herbs. Allow to cool.

Add in vitamin E oil and essential oils. Whip with a hand mixer for 10 minutes or until consistency is fluffy. If the butter is too runny, allow to cool in the fridge for 5 minutes before whipping again. Transfer to a glass jar. Apply to clean skin.

Homemade Facial Moisturizer

Ingredients:

4 Tbsp. aloe vera juice

1 tsp. vegetable glycerine

6 drops jojoba oil

¼ tsp. almond oil

Instructions:

Combine all ingredients in a 3 oz. bottle. Shake gently to mix. Shake before each use. Apply a few drops to skin, massaging in with fingertips.

Moisturizing Facial Oil

Ingredients:

2 Tbsp. hemp seed oil

5 drops carrot seed oil

5 drops palmarosa oil

Instructions:

Mix ingredients together and funnel into a small, dark glass bottle. Place lid tightly on bottle and shake to blend well. After cleansing skin, apply 2-3 drops to fingertips and massage into face gently.

Balancing Moisturizer

1 C. aloe vera gel (not juice)

¾ oz. beeswax pastilles

¼ C. coconut oil

¼ C. almond oil

10 drops sweet orange essential oil

2 drops tea tree oil

Instructions:

Using a double boiler, warm almond oil. Add beeswax and coconut oil and allow to melt together. Pour mixture into blender and leave to cool completely for 1 ½-2 hours (this prevents separation later). Mix orange and tea tree oils into the aloe vera gel. Turn blender on low and slowly add aloe. Continue until liquid thickens into a fluffy, whipped cream texture. Transfer to container with lid. Apply to freshly cleansed skin.

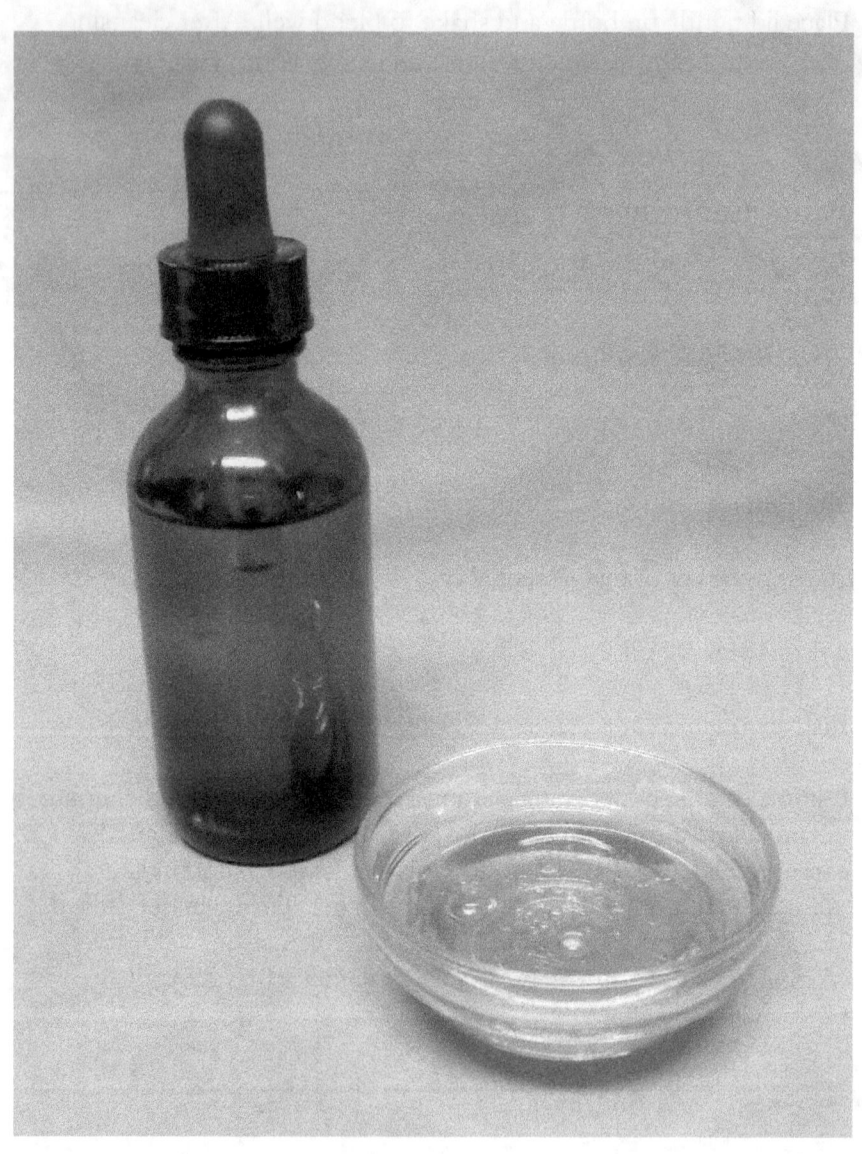

EYES

Green Tea Treatment (to reduce puffiness)

Ingredients:

2 green tea bags (***with*** caffeine)

Instructions:

Steep tea bags in hot water for 5 minutes. Squeeze out excess liquid and place tea bags in refrigerator for half an hour. Recline in a comfortable position and place over eyes for 10-15 minutes.

Parsley Eye Mask (to erase dark circles)

Ingredients:

1 handful of parsley

½ tsp. olive oil

1 Tbsp. hot water

Instructions:

Finely chop parsley and use a mortar and pestle to grind and crush leaves. Add olive oil and water, mixing thoroughly to form a thin paste. Wait a few minutes for mixture to cool and use cotton pads to soak up excess fluid. Recline somewhere comfortable and apply pads to the under eye area for 10-15 minutes. Rinse away excess gently and apply a thin layer of coconut oil or other natural moisturizer. Repeat one to three times per week for best results.

Soothing Cucumber Eye Gel

Ingredients:

4 oz. aloe vera gel

1/2 large cucumber, washed, peeled, and cut into cubes

Instructions:

Place cucumber in a blender and liquify. Strain 2 Tbsp. cucumber juice through cheesecloth into a glass jar. Add aloe vera gel and stir thoroughly to mix well. Chill before using. Apply under and around eyes nightly Store in refrigerator.

Eye Makeup Remover

Ingredients:

1 Tbsp. almond oil

1 Tbsp. coconut oil

1 Tbsp. olive oil

Instructions:

Combine all ingredients in a glass jar. Dip a cotton ball into oil. Sweep gently over eye area to remove cosmetics. Rinse.

Nourishing Eye Cream

Ingredients:

2 Tbsp. coconut oil

2 Tbsp. sweet almond oil

2 Tbsp. vitamin E oil

Instructions:

Mix all ingredients in a small bowl. Transfer to glass jar. Apply to cleansed skin with Q-tip. Pat into eye area gently with ring finger.

Dark Circle Fading Treatments

Ingredients:

2 chamomile teabags, steeped in water and squeezed out

OR

2 slices fresh cucumber, chilled

OR

2 slices red potato, chilled

Instructions:

Place on eyes, making sure to cover dark areas underneath. Recline and relax for 10 minutes. Remove treatment, rinse with cool water, pat dry and apply eye cream or oil.

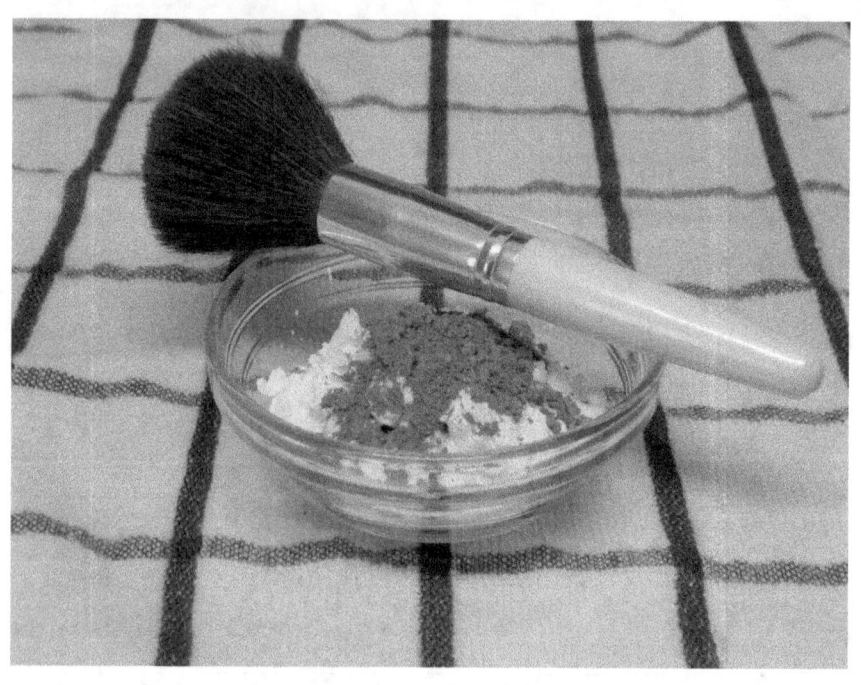

POWDERS

Cinnamon Body Dust

Ingredients:

¼ C. cornstarch

¼ C. rice flour

1 Tbsp. cinnamon powder

Instructions:

Mix all ingredients with a whisk. Pour powder into a glass jelly jar. Punch holes in lid to make a shaker. Shake powder on your skin after a shower, in your lingerie drawer or over bed linens.

Foundation Powder Make-up

(This is now the *only* make-up I use...*love* it!)

Instructions:

½ C. cornstarch

1 Tbsp. cocoa powder

1 tsp. ground cinnamon

Instructions:

Put cornstarch in medium size bowl. Gradually whisk in cocoa until you reach the level of your skin's natural shade. Add cinnamon to add warmth until you achieve the desired tone.

Apply with a powder puff and sweep off excess with a fluffy powder brush.

Bronzer

Ingredients:

½ Tbsp. arrowroot powder

½ Tbsp. cornstarch

1 Tbsp. cinnamon

1 Tbsp. cocoa

1 Tbsp. nutmeg

Instructions:

Combine all ingredients in a small glass jar. Shake well to blend. Apply with a fluff brush, being sure to tap off excess first. (for deeper bronze, add more cinnamon and nutmeg)

Shower Fresh Body Powder

Ingredients:

1 box cornstarch

15-20 drops tea tree oil

Instructions:

Place cornstarch in a lidded jar. Add tea tree oil and shake thoroughly for 2 minutes. Let sit one hour before using. Dust onto skin after or between showers for a fresh feeling!---

Natural Powder Blush

Ingredients:

1 Tbsp. arrowroot powder

½ tsp. corn starch

½ tsp. beetroot powder

Instructions:

In a small bowl, mix arrowroot and corn starch with a small whisk. Add beetroot powder and whisk to blend. Test on skin. If needed, add more arrowroot for more subtle results, or more beetroot for brighter blush. Store in reusable glass or plastic container.

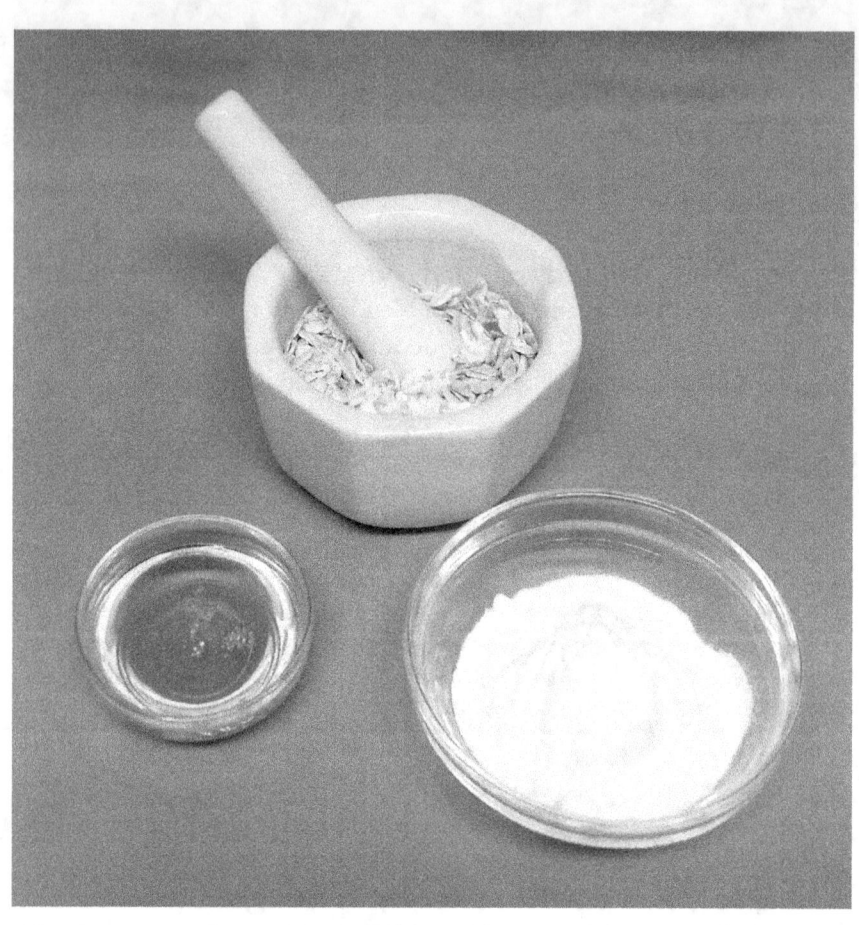

BODY SCRUBS

Are you one of those people who can't function until having consumed at least a pot of coffee? Does the aroma of freshly ground java beans make you tingle? Then the following recipes are a perfect fit for you! Note: Where the use of ground coffee is indicated, it is referring to straight from the can or grinder as opposed to after water has run through.

COFFEE SCRUBS

Wake Up Energy Scrub

Ingredients:

1/2 C. ground coffee

1/2 C. brown sugar

1/4 C. hot water

1/4 C. melted coconut oil (or sweet almond oil)

15 drops peppermint essential oil

Instructions:

Combine coffee grounds and sugar in a bowl. Add hot water, stir thoroughly and cool for 5 minutes or until mixture forms a paste. Add oils and mix well. Massage gently onto skin and rinse well. Pat skin dry.

Cinnamon Dolce Latte Scrub

Ingredients:

1/2 C. organic coconut oil

1 Tbsp. plain Greek yogurt

1 C. ground coffee

1/2 C. sugar

1/2 C. coarse sea salt

1/2 Tbsp. Cinnamon

1 Tbsp. Vanilla

Instructions:

Melt coconut oil and let it sit 5 minutes to cool slightly. Stir in yogurt. Add remaining ingredients and mix well. Apply to skin and massage gently. Rinse well.

Coconut Java Scrub

Ingredients:

1 C. ground coffee

1/2 C. dark brown sugar

1/2 C. sea salt

2/3 C. coconut oil

Instructions:

Melt coconut oil. Add in remaining ingredients and mix well. Apply to skin, massage gently, rinse thoroughly.

Vanilla Espresso Scrub

Ingredients:

¼ C. coconut oil, melted

¼ C. jojoba oil

½ C. brown sugar

½ C. ground coffee

5-8 drops pure vanilla

5-8 drops cinnamon essential oil

Instructions:

Mix all ingredients thoroughly in a bowl. Apply to clean, damp skin and massage gently for 30-60 seconds. Rinse completely and pat dry.

Coffee Scrub Cellulite Treatment

Ingredients:

1 C. sugar

1 C. caffeinated ground coffee

3/4 cup olive oil OR melted coconut oil

Spoonful water (adjust amount for desired consistency)

Instructions:

Mix ingredients in blender or with a hand mixer until smooth. Store in a glass jar. Apply after bathing while you are still in the shower. Massage into areas prone to cellulite in a gentle circular motion for at least two minutes. Rinse well with *cool* water, pat dry and follow with moisturizer.

Does the aroma of fresh fruit appeal to your senses? Are you soothed by the sweetness of strawberries or invigorated by the scent of citrus? Try one of these fruit based scrubs to refresh and smooth your skin with the sweetness of nature.

FRUIT SCRUBS

Zingy Citrus Scrub

Ingredients:

1 C. sugar

¼ C. coconut oil, melted

¼ cup jojoba oil

5 drops lemon essential oil

5 drops orange essential oil

Instructions:

Mix all ingredients together. Apply in shower after cleansing and massage gently onto skin. Rinse well. Pat dry. No need to use moisturizer since the natural oils in this scrub with leave a light protective barrier on the surface of your skin!

Sweet Berry Scrub

Ingredients:

¼ C. pureed blackberries, raspberries or strawberries

1 Tbsp. olive oil

1 Tbsp. coconut OR almond oil

1 Tbsp. vitamin E oil

2-3 Tbsp. of sugar (depending on how thick of a paste is desired)

Instructions:

Mix ingredients together. Apply after cleansing, gently massaging onto skin. Rinse well. Pat dry.

Energizing Coconut Lime Scrub

Ingredients:

¼ C. coconut oil, melted (may also use olive oil)

1 C. sugar

1 Tbsp. lime zest

Instructions:

Mix ingredients together. Apply after cleansing, gently massaging onto skin. Rinse well. Pat dry.

Pumpkin Pie Scrub

Ingredients:

1/2 C. pure canned pumpkin (*not* pie filling!)

1/2 C. brown sugar

1/4 Tsp. cinnamon

Sprinkle of nutmeg and/or ginger (optional)

Instructions:

Combine all ingredients and mix well. Apply to skin, scrub gently using circular motions. Rinse well and pat dry.

Honey Lemon Hand Scrub

Ingredients:

1 Tbsp. coconut oil

2 Tbsp. honey

1 Tbsp. lemon juice

1/4 C. celtic sea salt

1/4 C. sugar

Instructions:

Mix coconut oil and honey, stirring well. In a separate bowl, mix lemon juice, salt and sugar. Combine contents of both bowls together and mix well. Wash hands and then massage a nickel size amount of scrub into hands and fingers. Be gentle around cuticles! Rinse with warm water and pat dry. Repeat treatment weekly. ----------------------

Avocado Body Polish

Ingredients:

2 C. extra virgin olive oil *or* coconut oil

1/2 C. avocado oil

1/4 C. celtic sea salt

1 C. cornmeal

Instructions:

Stir oils together. Mix in salt and cornmeal a little at a time until a paste is formed. Apply after cleansing, gently massaging onto skin. Rinse well. Pat dry.

Perhaps teas and tinctures are more your style. These herb infused creations can help balance your skin as well as your mood.

HERBAL SCRUBS

Lavender Scrub

Ingredients:

1 C. sugar

1/3 C. celtic sea salt

1/2 C. coconut oil, melted

2 Tbsp. almond oil

1 Tbsp. vitamin E oil

5 drops lavender essential oil

Instructions:

Mix salt and sugar together. Add in oils and stir thoroughly. Add extra sugar or teaspoons of warm water to adjust texture until desired consistency is achieved.

Oatmeal & Lavender Body Polish

Ingredients:

1 C. oatmeal

1/4 C. dry powdered milk

1 Tbsp. cornmeal

10 drops lavender essential oil

1 Tbsp. warm water

Instructions:

Mix dry ingredients together. Add oil and water to form a paste. After cleansing, massage into skin in circular motion. Rinse well and pat skin dry. Store in glass jar and refrigerate for up to six months. (Scoop out desired amount and let sit until it reaches room temperature for a more comfortable application.)

Rosemary Lavender Skin Polish

Ingredients:

2 C. celtic sea salt

1/4 C. olive oil

3 Tbsp. dried lavender flowers, crushed

3 Tbsp. dried rosemary, crushed

3-5 drops lavender essential oil

Instructions:

Mix all ingredients together. After cleansing, apply with a gentle circular motion. Rinse well with warm water and pat skin dry.

Peppermint Pedi Foot Scrub

Ingredients:

2 C. sugar

1/4 cup almond oil or coconut oil

10 drops peppermint essential oil

5-10 drops pomegranate juice

Instructions:

Combine all ingredients. Soak feet in a warm bath for ten minutes. Apply scrub and thoroughly massage into feet and ankles, and in between toes. Rinse well and pat dry. Put on socks to allow the oils to penetrate *and* to protect against slipping on hard floors!

Gentle Vanilla Scrub

Ingredients:

1 C. white sugar

2 1/4 C. brown sugar

1/4 C. almond oil

4 Tbsp. vanilla

Instructions:

Mix sugars together. Add in almond oil and vanilla, mixing well. After cleansing, apply scrub with gentle pressure. Rinse and pat dry. (gentle enough to be used on the face, as well!)

Vanilla Honey & Chamomile Scrub

Ingredients:

1 C. brown sugar

1 Tbsp. loose chamomile tea leaves, crushed

¼ C. coconut oil

¼ C. jojoba OR almond oil

¼ C. honey, warmed

10 drops vanilla

Instructions:

Stir together sugar and tea leaves. Slowly add in oils, honey and vanilla and mix well. Cleanse, apply scrub and gently exfoliate. Scrub can be left on the skin for five-ten minutes as a balancing mask. Rinse well and pat dry.

Revitalizing Mint Body Polish

Ingredients:

1/4 C. brown sugar

2 Tbsp. coconut oil

2 Tbsp. honey

3-5 drops peppermint essential oil

Instructions:

Mix all ingredients together. After cleansing, apply to skin in a gentle circular motion. Rinse well and pat dry.

Invigorating Tea Tree Scrub

Ingredients:

2 Tbsp. olive oil

2 Tbsp. honey

2 Tbsp. plain Greek yogurt

3/4 C. sugar

5-8 drops tea tree essential oil

Instructions:

Mix oil, honey and yogurt together until smooth. Slowly add sugar until a paste is formed. Thoroughly stir in tea tree oil. Apply to clean skin and gently exfoliate. Rinse well and pat dry.

Sensitive Skin Soothing Scrub

Ingredients:

1 C. brown sugar

1 C. oatmeal

½ C. olive oil *or* coconut oil

½ C. plain Greek yogurt

Instructions:

Combine all ingredients and apply to clean skin. Gently exfoliate and rinse well with warm water. Follow with a cool rinse and pat skin dry.

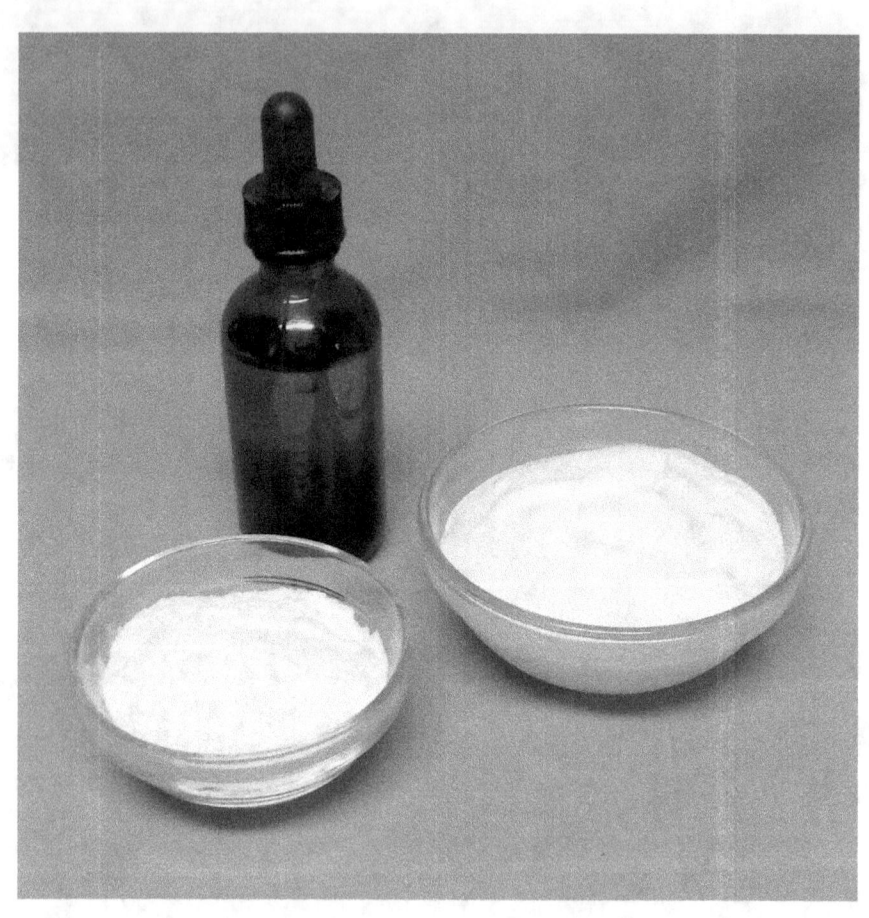

DEODORANTS

Recipe #1

Ingredients:

1/4 C. baking soda

1/4 C. arrowroot powder

1/3 C. cold coconut oil

5-10 drops essential oils (optional)

Instructions:

Mix baking soda and arrowroot powder in a bowl. Add cold coconut oil and cut into dry ingredients with a fork. If desired, add 8 drops of lavender or tea tree oil. Adjust amounts of oil and dry ingredients until desired texture is achieved. Store in a glass jar. Apply with fingertips and massage gently into underarms.

Recipe #2

Ingredients:

1/4 cup baking soda

1/4 cup arrow root powder *or* corn starch

5 Tbsp. coconut oil

Instructions:

Combine baking soda and arrow root powder in a bowl. Add half the oil and work into a paste. Gradually add the remaining oil and combine until desired consistency is achieved. Store in a glass jar.-----

Recipe #3

Ingredients:

1/3 C. coconut oil

1/4 C. baking soda

1/4 C. arrowroot powder

4 Tbsp. cornstarch

5-10 drops pure essential oil (orange, cinnamon, lavender, etc.)

Instructions:

Mix baking soda, cornstarch, and arrowroot powder in a bowl. Add coconut oil and cut into dry ingredients with a fork. Add your choice of essential oil and blend well. Adjust amount of coconut oil or baking soda to achieve desired consistency. In hot climates, it may be necessary to keep this in the refrigerator to prevent melting.

Recipe #4 (powder formula)

Ingredients:

1/4 C. baking soda

¼ C. cornstarch

10 drops tea tree oil

Instructions:

Whisk first two ingredients together and gradually add oil, continuing to whisk. Place in covered glass container. Apply with fluffy powder brush or puff.---

Recipe #5

Ingredients:

1/4 C. coconut oil

1 tsp. vitamin E oil

8-10 drops pure essential oil (tea tree, cinnamon, orange, lavender, etc.)

1/2 C. baking soda

1/2 C. corn starch

Instructions:

Mix together first three ingredients in a glass jar. Add in dry ingredients and mix thoroughly. Apply sparingly to underarms with fingertips.

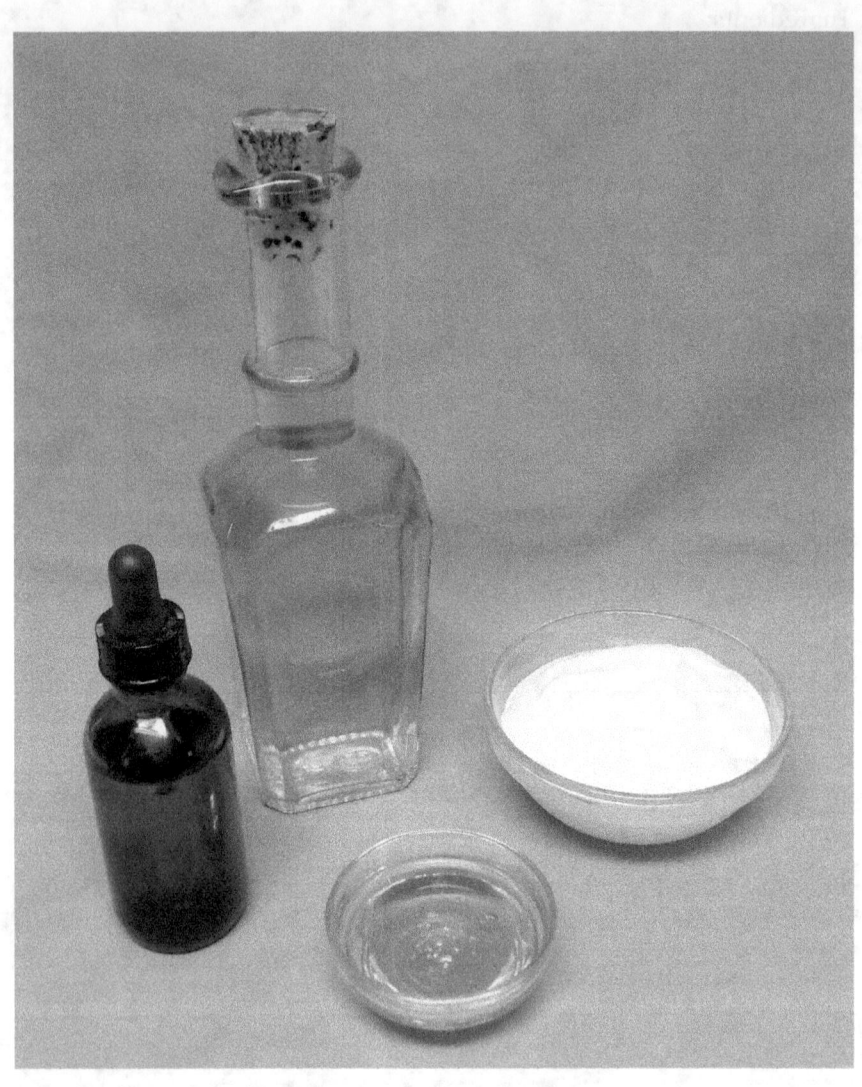

HAIR

DEEP CONDITIONING TREATMENT MASKS

Tropical Mask

Ingredients:

1 ripe avocado

1 ripe banana

3 Tbsp. coconut oil (melted)

1 Tbsp. raw honey

Instructions:

Place flesh of avocado and banana in blender with oil and honey, and pulse repeatedly until blended smooth. Apply to clean hair and massage into root area, working all the way to the ends. Pin up hair and cover with a shower cap or clear, plastic wrap. Let sit for 20 minutes, rinse, shampoo lightly and rinse again with cool water.

Tea Tree Treatment (for dry, itchy scalp)

Ingredients:

5 drops tea tree oil

1 Tbsp. olive oil

Instructions:

Mix oils in a small cup. Dip fingertips in oil and massage into scalp, concentrating on problem areas. Cover hair with a shower cap for 30 minutes, longer if desired. Shampoo lightly and condition ends.--------

Nourishing Moisturizing Mask (for dry hair)

Ingredients:

1 egg

1 Tbsp. vinegar

2 Tbsp. olive oil

3 Tbsp. raw honey

Instructions:

Mix all ingredients with a whisk. Apply to clean hair, and comb through from scalp to ends. Massage gently into scalp. Let sit for 15 minutes and rinse well with warm water.

Coconut Honey Mask (pre-shampoo)

Ingredients:

¼ C. coconut oil

1 tsp. raw honey

Instructions:

Microwave oil and honey for 30 seconds and stir to mix.

Work mixture into hair from scalp to ends, clip up hair and cover with shower cap for 15 minutes. Shampoo gently.

Coconut Oil Treatment

(I recommend this to my salon clients all the time…amazing results!)

Ingredients:

¼ - ½ C. organic virgin coconut oil (depending on length and thickness of hair)

Instructions:

Scoop a portion of oil with your fingers and apply to hair a section at a time. Continue until oil is gone and hair is saturated. Concentrate on ends and dry or damaged areas. Twist hair up on top of head and clip to hold in place. Cover with a shower cap or wrap head in plastic wrap to hold in body heat. Let sit for an hour. Alternatively, you can let sit for 30 minutes while warming with a blow dryer. Rinse well with warm water, shampoo and condition.

CONDITIONERS

Lemon Cream Conditioner

Ingredients:

2 Tbsp. lemon juice

1 egg yolk

1 Tbsp. raw honey

1 Tbsp. plain Greek yogurt

Instructions:

Mix all ingredients together, stirring well. Apply to freshly shampooed hair. Massage well through hair and let sit for 20 minutes. Rinse well with warm water.---

Honey Nut Conditioner

Ingredients:

½ C. raw honey

2 Tbsp. olive oil

1 Tbsp. almond oil

Instructions:

Mix all ingredients together, and apply liberally to freshly washed hair. Massage through hair, twist up and clip on top of your head. Cover hair with a shower cap or wrap with plastic wrap to hold in body heat. Let sit 30 minutes, and rinse thoroughly with warm water. Follow with a cool water rinse.

Nourishing Conditioner

Ingredients:

1 egg yolk

½ tsp. olive oil

¾ C. warm water

Instructions:

Beat egg yolk with a whisk. Add oil and continue to whisk. Finally, add water and whisk to combine. Apply to freshly washed hair and let sit 10 minutes. Rinse well with warm water.

Protein Conditioner

Ingredients:

1 egg white

¾ C. plain Greek yogurt

Instructions:

Beat egg white with a whisk until it foams. Spoon over yogurt and fold in. Apply to freshly washed hair and let sit for 15 minutes. Rinse well with warm water.

SHAMPOOS

No Rinse Shampoo

Ingredients:

1 Tbsp. cornstarch

4 Tbsp. water

1 Tbsp. white vinegar

Instructions:

Mix all ingredients in a spray bottle and shake to blend. Spray lightly at scalp and massage with fingers to absorb oil and dirt. Comb through and blow dry briefly.

Coconut Citrus Shampoo

Ingredients:

½ C. coconut milk

¾ C. all natural castile soap

15-20 drops orange essential oil

2 tsp. olive oil

Instructions:

Using a funnel, pour all ingredients in a bottle and shake well to blend. Shake well before each use.

Thickening Shampoo

Ingredients:

1 C. warm water

1 Tbsp. baking soda

¾ Tbsp. oat flour

¾ Tbsp. cornstarch

Instructions:

Mix all ingredients in a blender and pour through funnel into bottle or jar. Shake well before use.

Dry Shampoo

Ingredients:

½ C. baking soda

½ C. corn starch

8-10 drops lavender essential oil

Shaker bottle

Instructions:

Combine ingredients in a bowl and stir to mix well. Transfer to shaker bottle. To use, part hair into sections, sprinkling mixture at root area. Massage into scalp and hair with fingertips. Wait 5 minutes, bend forward to flip head upside down and gently brush out excess. Style as usual.

Super Clean Shampoo

Ingredients:

2 Tbsp. olive oil

1 egg

1 Tbsp. lemon juice

1 tsp. apple cider vinegar

10 drops tea tree oil

Instructions:

Combine all ingredients in a blender. Shampoo and rinse as usual.-----

SPRAYS

Detangling Spray

Ingredients:

4 oz. aloe vera juice

20 drops lavender essential oil

15 drops orange essential oil

5 drops rosemary essential oil

Instructions:

Combine ingredients in a spray bottle and shake well. Spray liberally through freshly washed hair, and comb through.

Sea Salt Texture Spray

Ingredients:

2 C. hot water

1 Tbsp. sea salt

1 Tbsp. coconut oil

Instructions:

Combine all ingredients in a spray bottle. Shake well. Spray onto damp hair. Twist or braid sections of hair and allow to air dry. When dry, lightly shake out hair with fingers being careful to not break down the texture.

Hair Spray

Ingredients:

2 oranges (for dry hair) *or* 2 lemons (for oily hair)

2 C. water

Instructions:

Chop fruit into small pieces. Place in a pot and add water. Boil until reduced by half. Cool solution, strain and funnel into spray bottle. Store in refrigerator.

MISCELANEOUS HAIR PRODUCTS

Natural Hair Gel

Ingredients:

1 C. filtered water

2 Tbsp. flax seeds

5 drops essential oil of your choice

1 tsp. aloe vera gel

Instructions:

Bring water to a boil. Stir in flax seeds, turn down to medium and simmer for between for 8 minutes. Strain out flax seeds and allow gel to cool. Stir in essential oil and aloe vera. Pour gel into a bottle and use a quarter size amount for hair. Massage in and comb through. Style as usual. Store gel in refrigerator.

ACV Clarifying Rinse (great for oily hair or product build up)

Ingredients:

¼ C. apple cider vinegar

1 C. filtered water

Instructions:

Shampoo hair as usual and rinse. Slowly pour mixture over hair and work through length with hands. Rinse well and feel the clean! Finish by applying a light conditioner to ends of hair. Rinse.

Scalp Scrub (for dandruff or dry scalp)

Ingredients:

2 Tbsp. shampoo

1 Tbsp. baking soda

Instructions:

Mix ingredients to form a paste. Work through hair, concentrating on root area. Massage scalp with fingertips to remove dead skin. Rinse well and condition.

Herbal Tea Rinse (to bring out natural highlights)

Ingredients:

1 gallon water

4 tea bags (chamomile for blonds, black tea for brunettes, red zinger for redheads)

Instructions:

Boil water and pour into a gallon pitcher. Add tea bags, and steep for five minutes. Allow tea to cool. Lean over the edge of the tub or sink and flip your hair so it hangs down. Slowly pour entire amount of tea over your hair and allow the excess to drip off. Blot ends lightly with paper towels and wrap hair up on top of your head, clipping it in place. Cover with a shower cap or plastic wrap and let sit 10-15 minutes. Rinse out, shampoo lightly, and condition as usual.

Anti-Frizz Serum

Ingredients:

4 oz. camellia oil

½ oz. castor oil

½ oz. avocado oil

20 drops essential oil of your choice

Instructions:

Combine all ingredients together and funnel into a glass bottle with a dropper. To use, place 3-5 drops in the palm of your hand. Rub between hands and work into ends of hair, gliding over mid-shaft of hair to reduce frizziness and add shine.

Lemon Rinse (for oily hair)

Ingredients:

½ C. lemon juice

½ C. brewed black tea

Instructions:

Combine ingredients in a measuring cup. Shampoo hair as usual and pour mixture over hair. Work through with fingers and rinse. Finish with a light conditioner on ends.

Cranberry Shine Booster

Ingredients:

16 oz. bottle cranberry juice

Instructions:

Shampoo as usual. Pour juice over hair and work through with fingers. Rinse.

Hair Growth Treatment

Ingredients:

1 tsp. raw honey

2 tsp. olive oil

2 tsp. coconut oil

½ avocado (mashed)

Instructions:

Mix all ingredients until smooth. Massage into dry hair and let sit for 15 minutes. Rinse out, shampoo and condition as usual.

Watercress Treatment (for oily hair)

Ingredients:

2 large handfuls fresh watercress

1 C. filtered water

1 Tbsp. lemon juice

Instructions:

Combine ingredients in blender. Place in saucepan and heat to boiling. Allow to boil for 10 minutes. Strain mixture and let the liquid cool. Shampoo as usual. Towel dry hair and pour mixture through tresses, working into scalp with fingertips. Let sit for 20 minutes. Rinse and condition ends of hair.

Shine Serum

Ingredients:

A few drops coconut oil

Instructions:

Once hair is dry and you have curled or straightened it, rub oil between hands and apply to mid-shaft of hair, working down to ends. Don't use too much or the hair will end up greasy instead of shiny. This is also a fantastic way to control frizz and give your hair an added dose of moisture that lasts all day.

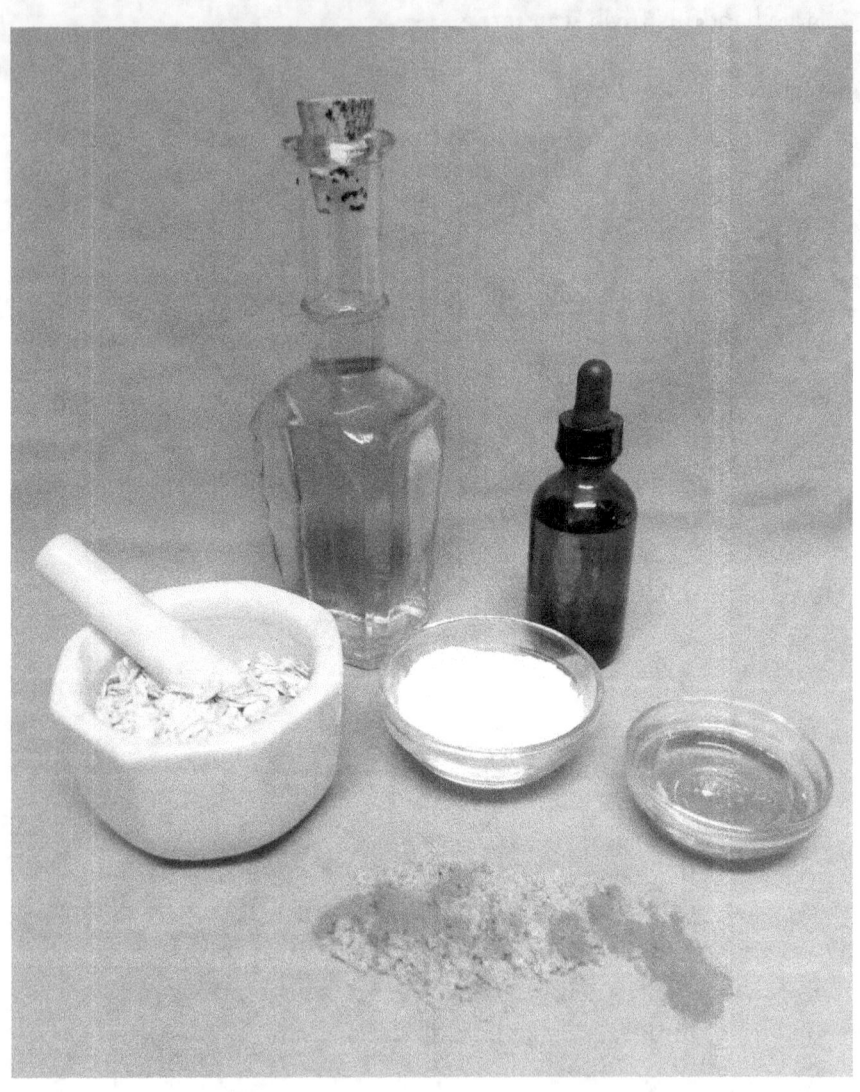

MISCELLANEOUS

Sunburn Spritz

Ingredients:

½ C. aloe vera gel

15 drops lavender essential oil

5 drops peppermint essential oil

10 drops vitamin E oil

Instructions:

Pour ingredients into a spray bottle. Secure top and shake vigorously to blend. Spray on sunburned skin as needed for relief. Store in refrigerator.

Dark Spot Treatments

(for oily skin)

Ingredients:

lemon juice

Instructions:

After cleansing skin, apply a few drops of lemon juice to dark spots with a cotton swab. Allow to air dry before using any other products.

(for dry or sensitive skin)

Ingredients:

aloe vera juice

Instructions:

After cleansing skin, apply a few drops of aloe vera juice to dark spots with a cotton swab. Wait 45 minutes before applying any other products.

Soft Feet Solution

Ingredients:

2 C. apple cider vinegar

warm water

Instructions:

Fill a large basin with vinegar and water and place on the floor in front of a comfortable chair. Sit down and place feet in solution. Soak for 20 minutes. Pat dry and apply moisturizer.

Honey Rose Soak

Ingredients:

2 C. whole milk

½ C. raw honey

5 drops rose essential oil

Instructions:

Stir together milk, honey, and rose oil. Pour slowly into bath tub full of warm water. Soak in bath for 20 minutes or until water cools for soft, smooth skin.---

Callus Remover

Ingredients:

2 Tbsp. baking soda

3 Tbsp. brown sugar

8 drops lavender essential oil

Instructions:

Take a warm bath or shower to pre-soften skin. Mix ingredients together, adding a few drops of water at a time to form a paste. Scrub feet with mixture, concentrating on callused areas. Rinse well, pat dry and slather on a thick application of coconut oil (or natural moisturizer of choice). Put on cotton socks so moisture absorbs deep into tissue.

Stretch Mark Miracle Oil

Ingredients:

¼ C. coconut oil

2 Tbsp. cocoa butter

2 tsp. sweet almond oil

Instructions:

In heavy saucepan over low heat, warm ingredients. Stir until well blended and clear. Cool. Store in wide mouth jar. Massage into skin morning and evening.

Peppermint Foot Rub

Ingredients:

2 Tbsp. coconut oil (or another oil of your choice... jojoba, almond, etc.)

1 tsp. white vinegar

1/2 tsp. peppermint essential oil

Instructions:

Pour ingredients into glass jar and stir to blend. Apply to clean, dry feet, massaging with firm pressure. Elevate legs and feet and relax for 20 minutes. Finish by putting on cotton socks to allow oils to penetrate deeply into tissue.

Natural Self Tanner

Ingredients:

4 tea bags (plain, black tea)

2 C. water

Instructions:

Bring water to a boil. Steep tea bags for 15 minutes and allow to cool. Remove bags and pour tea into a spray bottle. In the shower, cleanse and exfoliate skin. Rinse well and dry off completely. Remain in the shower to catch the drips and spray mixture evenly over body, using a lighter mist on areas that tend to be drier such as elbows, knees and heels. Air dry and repeat with a second application. For darker results, continue the cycle of application with dry time in between. NOTE: Be sure that your skin is totally dry before getting dressed, or the tea may stain your clothes!---

Peppermint Toothpaste

Ingredients:

2/3 C. baking soda

1 tsp. fine sea salt

½ packet stevia powder

2 Tbsp. coconut oil

20 drops peppermint essential oil

Instructions:

In a small bowl, mix together baking soda, salt and stevia powder. Using a fork, cut in coconut oil while it is in a semi-solid state. Add peppermint oil and stir to blend completely. Transfer to a glass jar with a lid (baby food jars work great!) To use, wet toothbrush under warm water and dip brush into paste, picking up about a pea size amount. Brush as usual. NOTE: If more than one person will be using this toothpaste, give each individual their own jar to prevent transfer of bacteria.

So Silky Shaving Solution

Ingredients:

2 C. sugar

¾ C. coconut oil OR olive oil

¼ C. lemon juice

8 drops tea tree oil

Instructions:

Mix ingredients in a bowl or jar, stirring thoroughly to blend. Take a shower or bath to pre-soften skin. Apply mixture to legs and massage to exfoliate skin. Rinse well and then shave. Repeat steps for an ultra-smoothing effect. After shaving, rinse with warm water, then cool. No need to use moisturizer as the oils in the mixture will leave a thin coating on your skin. WARNING! There may also be an oily film on the shower/tub floor as well, so clean it up to avoid a fall from the slipperiness.

Lash Thickener

Ingredients:

1 tsp. castor oil

½ tsp. vitamin E oil

¼ tsp. aloe vera gel

Instructions:

Blend ingredients in a small glass container with a lid. Using a clean mascara wand, apply mixture to lashes on a nightly basis.

All Natural Sunscreen

Ingredients:

¼ C. aloe vera gel

¼ C. sesame oil OR coconut oil

1 tsp. vitamin E oil

20 drops lavender essential oil

Instructions:

Stir ingredients together in a bowl to blend completely. Transfer to a bottle. Apply before sun exposure, re-applying every 2-3 hours or after swimming/sweating.

Swelling Relief Oil (for feet, ankles & legs)

Ingredients:

2 Tbsp. coconut oil (melted)

2 drops grapefruit essential oil

2 drops lemongrass essential oil

2 drops cypress essential oil

Instructions:

Mix ingredients. Scoop some out, rubbing hands together to coat palms. Massage gently into feet and ankles. Move upwards on legs with long sweeping motions. Relax and elevate feet and legs for 30 minutes.

Natural Teeth Whitening

Ingredients:

1 capsule activated charcoal powder

1 Tbsp. hydrogen peroxide

water

Instructions:

Wet your toothbrush under running water. Break open capsule and sprinkle charcoal onto toothbrush. Brush teeth in a gentle, circular motion for 2 minutes. Spit out excess and rinse your mouth out with water. Sip peroxide into mouth (do *NOT* swallow!) and swish around and through teeth for at least 30 seconds. Spit and rinse mouth out with water several times. WARNING! Although it whitens teeth, charcoal will stain other things! Clean your toothbrush and sink immediately and be careful to not get it on your clothing.

Blemish Treatment

Ingredients:

lavender essential oil

Instructions:

After cleansing skin, apply a drop or two of lavender oil to blemish with a cotton swab. Repeat 2-3 times daily to speed up the healing process.

ABOUT THE AUTHOR

L. Joy Douglas is the author of several inspirational books
which can be found on Amazon.com
or through her personal web site at
www.joy4rain.wix.com/ljoydouglas.
Along with a passion for writing, she has been using her creativity
within the beauty industry since 1990.
The release of this book marks the official blending together
of the two things that have been her lifelong inspiration;
making people beautiful and creating beauty with words.